Ketogenic Diet

Lose Weight, Avoid Mistakes, And Feel Amazing!

TABLE OF CONTENTS

Introduction

Thank you for purchasing the book, *Ketogenic: Lose Weight, Avoid Mistakes, and Feel Amazing*!

Most people had begun to gather interest in the ketogenic diet a couple of years ago. This was because they had gained the information that they would lose weight quicker than most other diets. This book would try to answer most of the questions that you have about the diet.

The ketogenic diet has always been encircled by dispute at all times. People who have promoted the ketogenic diet claim that the diet is magical when compared to its opponents. This is due to the misconceptions that most people have about the diet. But, the reality exists somewhere in between all the misconceptions. But, there are drawbacks and advantages of the diet that are discussed thoroughly in the book that will help you understand how you can make the diet work for you.

There are guidelines in the book that will help you work through your diet when you begin. You will have to remember that a person who performs a lot of exercise will need to follow a diet that is slightly different since they will need to have a good amount of carbohydrates unlike other diets. There is one other diet apart from the traditional ketogenic diet that allows the consumption of carbohydrates with exercise.

This book acts as a guide for a person who is beginning the ketogenic diet. This book includes information for both the general public and the athletes and bodybuilders who perform a lot of exercise. The book also leaves you with a number of recipes that are mouthwatering! At the end of the book, you have been given a sample 7-day plan. You could use this plan to test whether or not you will be able to follow the ketogenic diet.

Thank you for purchasing the book. I hope it helps you!

Chapter 1:
An Introduction to the Ketogenic Diet

There are a lot of readers who are not familiar with the basics of the ketogenic diet. This chapter deals with some of the common ideas about the ketogenic diet and will also help you in defining certain terms. The basic definition is that the ketogenic diet is one that makes the liver produce ketone bodies that ensures that your body moves away from the usage of glucose to the use of the fat in order to provide you with energy.

To be very specific, when you are on a ketogenic diet, you will have to consume a lesser number of carbohydrates. You will need to maintain the consumption below a certain point, preferably 100 grams a day. This would imply that you would have to adapt in order to keep yourself healthy and fit. You could consume any quantity of protein or fat depending on your aims. But, your diet turns ketogenic depending on the presence or absence of carbohydrates.

The metabolism and the ketogenic diet

Every standard diet has a proper mix of carbohydrates, fats and protein. But, when you stop providing your body with carbohydrates, you are depleting the reserves that your body has rapidly. It is because of this that your body will have to look for a different way to provide you with energy. One such alternative is the fat that has been stored in your body in the form of acids. Your tissues will begin to use this fat to fuel your body with energy. But, not every organ can use these fatty acids. Instead, they use the ketone bodies that are released by the liver.

There are times when the fatty acids are not broken down well in your liver. The by – products of this partial breakdown are the ketone bodies. They are not carbohydrates and work as fuel for many tissues including the brain. When you stop consuming carbohydrates, your body produces more ketone bodies, which then flow into the blood stream leading to ketosis that is a metabolic state. There will also be a decrease in the production and the utilization of glucose. When ketosis occurs, your body will begin to decrease the protein in your body to provide you with energy. There are a lot of people who use the ketogenic diet to lose the fat in their body while keeping enough body mass to have a lean body.

Hormones and the ketogenic diet

As mentioned previously, the ketogenic diet requires your body to adapt to a few changes. The diet results in a change in the levels of the hormones glucagon and insulin. Insulin is a hormone that helps in moving the nutrients in the blood stream to the tissues that require those nutrients – it works as a storage hormone. For instance, insulin helps in storing glucose in the muscles in the form of glycogen. Glucagon is a hormone that helps in stimulating your body to break down the glycogen that has been stored by the muscles, most often in the liver, in order to give your body sufficient amount of glucose.

When you stop consuming carbohydrates, the level of insulin in your body begins to decrease while the level of glucagon in your body begins to increase. This immediately increases the fatty acids that are released from the fat cells in your body that are broken down in the liver. This process helps in the production of the ketone bodies that lead to ketosis. There are a lot of other hormones that are affected in the process. But, these hormones help in shifting the focus away from carbohydrates to the fats.

Exercise and the ketogenic diet

Like every other diet, you will find that the effects of the ketogenic diet are visible and will last only when you exercise. But, when you keep your body from consuming too many carbohydrates, you will find yourself unable to perform a good level of exercise. This is why a person who is an athlete or a bodybuilder must ensure that he integrates carbohydrates into the diet without affecting the process of ketosis. There is a diet that has been described in the book that helps you incorporate carbohydrates in your diet some time before or after you perform your exercise.

The benefits of the ketogenic diet

There are a lot of benefits that the ketogenic diet provides. This section covers a few of them.

Reduced appetite

The ketogenic diet is one where you consume a lot of proteins. It is well known that proteins are quite filling and so, you will not feel hungry as often. This therefore will cause you to eat less and also feel less hungry. However, that will not mean you will feel weak or incapable of carrying out your day-to-day activities. You will feel just as energetic as you always have! This is a good thing since you will find yourself energetic throughout the day on account of the fatty acids being burnt in your body. When you are on a diet, you often find yourself craving for food. This is one of the most important reasons behind why a person feels depressed and gives up on the diet that he is following. The best thing that happens to you when you eat a low carb diet is that you will find your appetite decreasing. There are a few studies that have concluded that a person eating higher amounts of fat and protein and lower amounts of carbohydrates will consume a less amount of calories.

Loss of weight

The easiest way to lose weight when on a diet is by cutting the amount of carbohydrates that you consume. There have been quite a few studies that have been conducted which conclude the statement made above. The main reason behind this is that when you are on a low carbohydrate diet, your body will start losing the water that is found in excess in the body. This would lower the insulin levels in the body that would then lead to the loss of excess sodium from the body that would result in a rapid loss of weight in a week or two. There are studies that have said that a person on a low fat diet tends to lose weight slower than a person on a low carbohydrate diet since he will stop feeling too hungry.

When a person is on a low carbohydrate diet, he will lose weight for the first six months but soon the weight he lost would be catching up to him since he would have quit the diet. This is because of the fact that human beings have always viewed diets as boring. But, if you want to lose weight, it is good to view the ketogenic diet as a lifestyle and not a diet! This is the only way by which you will be able to stick to the diet. When you are on the ketogenic diet, you also have the option to add healthy carbohydrates into your diet when you have reached the ideal weight for your stature.

You will also be forced to consume a lot of water while on the diet. This water will aid in melting or dissolving the fat and carrying it out of the body. Therefore, you will start feeling quite light. You will not have to put in too many efforts towards losing the excess fat that remains when you turn skinny. The water will do the job for you. It will also kick start your metabolic activities. It will increase your metabolic rate and you will digest food better. So, it will not be just a temporary process and you will have the chance to stave off excess weight gain for good!

Loss of abdominal fat

People have the notion that if they start exercise, they will be able to lose fat in different parts of the body at the same time! They forget that the fat in the different muscles in the body is not the same! Your health is determined by how much of fat has been stored in which part of your body. But, there are two types of fat that you should know about – the visceral fat that is found in the abdomen and the subcutaneous fat that is found under the skin. The former is what is dangerous to your health since the fat surrounds itself around your organs.

When you have a lot of fat in your abdominal cavity, you will find yourself prone to inflammation. Due to this, you will also turn your body into being resistant against insulin. The visceral fat has found to be the cause of numerous metabolic diseases in most countries! When you are on a low carbohydrate diet, you will find that you have a greater chance of reducing the amount of fat in your abdominal region. The fat that is used most often to provide you with energy comes from your abdominal cavity! This would eventually reduce the risk of heart disease and Type II diabetes.

Reduced Levels of blood sugar

This is the best benefit since this also reduces the chances of procuring Type II diabetes and if you have it, you will be able to maintain the level of insulin in your body due to the diet.

When you eat carbohydrates, your body breaks them down into smaller sugars, most often glucose, in your digestive tract. The simple sugars then enter the bloodstream and spike the level of sugar in your blood. It is toxic to have high levels of sugar in your blood. To reduce the sugar level, your body produces insulin, which then indicates to the cells that the glucose has to either be stored in them or be used by them to provide your body with energy. When people are healthy, the insulin in their body helps in reducing the level of sugar in the blood that will help in protecting us from any harm.

There are many people who have a problem against this system. They are resistant to insulin, which implies that the cells do not find any insulin in their body. This makes it very difficult to transfer the sugar from the blood to the cells. This leads to Type II diabetes that most people in this generation are prone to having. This type of diabetes occurs when your body stops secreting the right amount of insulin to reduce the level of sugar in the blood when you have finished your meals.

You will find that the simplest solution to this problem is to cut the number of carbohydrates you consume on a regular basis. When you cut down on the carbohydrates, you will find that the level of blood sugar and insulin reduce drastically. A study was conducted to test whether the diet would benefit the million people out there who are suffering from diabetes. It was found that 95.2% of the people had managed to eliminate or lower the medication to lower their glucose levels while on the ketogenic diet. If you have Type II diabetes, it would be best for you to meet your doctor before you reduce your intake of carbohydrates. This is required to ensure that you do not suffer from hypoglycemia.

Great hair, skin

Proteins are vital for the body. They aid in strengthening your hair and also skin cells. The consumption of water will help in removing toxins from your body, which will reflect on your skin. You will see that your skin has cleared up and it is glowing. The diet will also help in increasing your confidence, as you will have great health.

Chapter 2:
What to Do On the Diet

The ketogenic diet is great for all those that wish to lose weight and remain slim for life. As you know, there are many low carb diets to pick from such as the Atkins diet and the paleo diet.

Here, we will look at some things that you can do on the diet to help it work better.

Prepare yourself

It would be a great idea for you to prepare yourself mentally. Many times, we think we are ready for a diet but our minds will actually not allow us to pursue it. If you want to prevent yourself from going back on your diet owing to a rebelling mind, then it is best that you prepare yourself for the road ahead. You have to tell yourself to be prepared for everything the diet puts your way and embrace it. Only then will you be able to successfully take up and stick with the diet.

Make a plan

Next, you have to devise a plan for the diet. Try to create a timetable of sorts and then go about following it. Not many people realize that it is important to not only plan your diet but also make a list of daily things that you should do for it. You can create a schedule that helps you know when to eat, when to exercise, when to drink water etc. You can create the list and maintain a hard copy of it and also a soft copy that you can pull out whenever and read from.

Time your intake

There is a golden rule about low carb diets that you should know and use to your advantage. As you already know, it is important for people to consume a little carbohydrate on a daily basis in order to remain fit and energetic. But what they don't realize is that it is possible to trick the body into believing that no carbs were taken in. this will help it burn the carbs away rather easily. The trick is to consume the carbs right before an exercise routine. The body will have the capacity to burn the carbs in a better way if you do so. You must also avoid consuming any carbs before bedtime, as your body might not digest it well enough.

Increase the fiber

It is best for you to increase the fiber in your diet. As you know, fiber plays a very important role in any diet, let alone the low carb diet. Fiber is a food element that is not digested by the body at all. But it puts in a lot of effort to break it down thereby exercising your digestive organs. There are many sources of fiber that you consume. However, you must stay away from glutinous foods even if they are loaded with fiber. Look for the best alternatives.

Consume fats

Do not make the mistake of avoiding fats when you are on the low carb diet. Many wonder why the diet allows fats to be consumed, especially when people are trying to lose weight. Fats that you consume will not usually get stored as fat in your body. In fact, your body will start putting in extra effort to break it down and so; it is a great idea for you to incorporate fat in your diet. Adding in a teaspoon of butter or ghee to your everyday foods will prove to be quite beneficial to your diet.

Drink water

It is important for you to remain as hydrated as possible in order to avoid any side effects of the diet. Try to consume at least 8 glasses of water a day. By replenishing your body and cells, you will be able to nourish it thoroughly. If you think it is a bit too boring to consume plain water, then you can try adding in a few cut fruits to it to make fruit infused water. The goal is to remain as hydrated as possible and aiding your digestive system in breaking down the different foods that you consume.

Consume supplements

When it comes to diets, there will always be one nutrient or the other that the body will not be able to acquire in the right proportion. This can be a problem if you wish to remain healthy. You will have to ensure that you are getting all the right nutrients and are able to lead a healthy life. The ketogenic diet also causes the body to not avail some important nutrients. For this, you will have to consume supplements that will help in adding these nutrients to your body. What you will need to consume will be determined by your physician and you will have to follow his or her instructions.

Cheat meals

It is important for any dieter to consume a few cheat meals. These refer to meals that you consume to take a break from your diet. These will act, as rewards that will help you remain motivated. The cheat meals can be anything that you like such as pizza or burger. You have to pre-decide on a meal that will act as your cheat meal. You have to determine the time as well as it will help you prepare for the meal and remain ready with it to be consumed.

Measure progress

It is important that you measure your progress with the diet. This means that you should know how the diet is working for you. If you don't know whether it is working and if you are slimming down, then there is no point in dieting and you might as well stop with it. So, the best thing is to maintain a journal and write down your experiences with the diet. You will have to measure your weight from time to time and see if you have scaled down. That is the best way to check the diet's efficacy.

Remain patient

Patience is important with any diet. You should have faith in it and know that it will work for you. Try to appreciate your body the way it is and tell yourself that you will love it no matter what. The best thing is to maintain a journal and write down a few goals that you will have to pursue in order to make a success out of your diet. The goals will help you stay on track and allow you in remaining put with the diet for a long time!

These are some of the right things that you can do with the ketogenic diet in order to stick with it.

Chapter 3:
What Not to Do On the Diet

As is with most things in life, there are a few things that you must not do on the ketogenic diet. Here is a list of things that you must avoid.

Stress yourself

To start with, do not stress yourself out. Stress is a common worry these days given the type of hectic lives that people lead. It is common for people to feel tensed and that leads to stress and anxiety. If you don't have a peace of mind, then your diet will not work for you. You might end up consuming foods that are prohibited by the diet and also cause the stress to reverse the effects of the diet. So, it is best that you remain as calm as possible. You can take up activities that will help you with the process. Some of it includes exercising and meditating, both of which will calm you down.

Lose sleep

It is important for your body to rejuvenate and replenish in order to work properly. So, you must give it ample rest. Not sleeping enough will cause you to reverse the effects of the diet. You have to therefore try and sleep for at least 8 hours a day. Try hitting the bed an hour early so that you give yourself enough time to fall asleep. You have to try and create an ideal setting to fall asleep like dim the lights, play light music, burn aroma candles etc. These will help you sleep fast and better.

Be negative

You must not be negative and always have a positive mindset. You must invest faith in the diet and be confident that it will help you lose weight and remain slim. If you always question whether or not the diet will work for you then you will end up making it difficult. Remember that the mind and body are connected at a very deep level and your body will work according to your mind's directions.

Cut out nutrients

Many times, in a bid to follow a strict diet, people end up cutting out vital nutrients from it. They will not realize that they have cut out important nutrients while trying to remain within the limits set out by the diet. This can be a bad thing, especially if you are following the ketogenic diet. Even a proper low carb diet will end up denying your body a few vital nutrients and if you further cut them out then it will only get worse. So, it is important that you eat nutritious meals even while following the low carb diet.

Eat too many calories

As was mentioned earlier, it is fine for you to consume a meal that has fats in it, but that does not mean you start consuming too many calories. There can be many little things in your diet that will increase the amount of calories. These can include nuts, fats and processed sugars from junk foods. You have to try and count the calories in your meals. It will be a little difficult in the beginning but will get better with time. You will know to keep track of all the calories that you will consume in a day.

Not exercise

As is with any diet, you have to exercise in order to lose your excess weight. You cannot lose your extra weight soon enough if you rely on the diet alone. The diet will help you shed extra pounds no doubt but you should also take up an exercise routine that will allow the lost weight to not return back. The exercise routine need not be too rigid. You can work with a personal trainer to come up with the routine to follow.

Celebrate too much

It was said before that it is fine for you to consume a cheat meal every now and then. This will help you remain focused and on track with your diet. However, you must not consume too many cheat meals. You should limit it to just a few meals a month. There is no point in eating foods that the diet prohibits. You will end up reversing its effect on your body. You can pre-determine the times for the cheat meals in order to prepare for them. You might also know to eat less before your cheat meal.

Pressurize yourself

Do not pressurize yourself too much to lose weight fast. You have to remain patient. It is not advisable to lose a lot of weight too soon. You have to set reasonable goals to lose weight. You have to ask your physician about it. Start by setting out reasonable goals and then pursue it one after the other.

Peer pressure

Sometimes, people start getting affected by what others have to say. You should try and remain unaffected by what others have to say about your diet. You should remain indifferent to it and remain focused on the task at hand.

Chapter 4:
Some Side Effects to Expect with the Ketogenic Diet

There can be a few side effects that the ketogenic diet can cause and they are mentioned as under.

Headache/ dizziness

Headache and dizziness is a very common aspect that is associated with the ketogenic diet. It usually occurs when a lot of the salt and minerals are removed from the body owing to the loss of water. The process of ketosis results in the elimination of water from the body, which takes out the salts and minerals as well. For this, you can try consuming more water a day in order to replenish all that was lost from the body.

Urination

It is also quite common for a person to urinate often when on the ketogenic diet. This is mainly because the diet causes excess water to be removed from the body. This is either eliminated through sweating or through urination. But don't be under the impression that consuming less water will help you solve the issue. That is not the right way to go about it and you must not cut down on the amount of water that you consume. You should keep it at regular levels and in fact have more in order to make up for the lost water.

Diarrhea

Diarrhea is said to be caused during the ketogenic diet. As you know, the body goes through a lot of diet change, which can cause your digestive system to go for a toss. The excess elimination of water from the body might also cause you to experience lose motions. For this, you can consume foods that are anti-diarrheal. You can also speak with your physician and ask for a suggestion that will help you beat your diarrhea and up your health.

Constipation

The ketogenic diet might also cause constipation. The consumption of too many proteins in the diet can sometimes cause you to feel constipated. For this, you can consume some natural laxatives. The laxatives might help with motions. You can ask for the best one and consume it. You must also increase your water intake as that will help with the process. You must also increase the fiber in your food as that too will help in fixing your constipation problem.

Weakness

Weakness is another complaint that people have with the ketogenic diet. In fact, it is generally associated with all types of diets. Not consuming enough nutrients and also the lack of sugar can cause you to feel weak. For this, you have to eat regular meals and consume fruits and vegetables. You should also drink enough water and that will help you stave off the weakness. You should also consume foods that are rich in multi vitamins. It is a must for you to consume supplements on a regular basis, as that will help you stave off weaknesses.

Muscle pain

Muscle pain is often associated with the ketogenic diet. This generally comes about owing to the dietary changes. It might not be limited to muscle pain alone and might also extend to joints. You might also experience cramps, which will make you quite uncomfortable. This generally happens as soon as you wake up or while retiring to bed. It might also happen when you take up an arduous activity. One good way to deal with this issue is by consuming foods that are rich in natural oils. It can be acquired through nuts, fish etc. You can also indulge in regular exercise, which will aid in reducing the muscle and joint pain.

Mood swings

Some people complain of mood swings. The elimination of essential minerals and other nutrients can cause people to experience several mood swings. They might cause people to feel happy one minute and angry the next. This is generally seen as being quite annoying. And although most people don't realize that their diet is causing it and start blaming other things for it. One way of dealing with this is by increasing the fiber content in your diet. That will aid in digestion and also elimination of the excess food in your body and improve your mood considerably. You will feel much better after increasing fiber and also other vital nutrients in your food.

Sugar cravings

Since the low carb diet causes a person to cut down on the amount of carbs/ sugars that are consumed, he or she will start craving sugar. This is only natural. But it would be useless to give into it, as that will cause you to go back on your diet. You will end up exposing your body to sugar once again. Instead, you should try and control yourself as much as possible. The craving will automatically disappear after a while and you will not feel like consuming any sugar-laden foods again.

Insomnia

Some people on the ketogenic diet complain about insomnia or lack of sleep. Insomnia is generally caused when there is an imbalance of the serotonin levels in the brain. Some diets can cause the same and so, it is best that you work on raising the level of serotonin in your brain. You can exercise and increase the levels. You will feel much better and be able to sleep better.

Bad breath

Bad breath is quite common amongst those that take up the ketogenic diet. The process of ketosis induces bad breath and should not be a major cause of concern. However, it is quite easy for you to get rid of your bad breath. You can brush your teeth more often and also clean your tongue. You can consume foods that help in cutting out bad breath such as mint leaves and basil leaves. Consume 10 leaves every morning and your bad breath issue will be dealt with.

These are some of the common side effects associated with the ketogenic diet.

Chapter 5:
Some Things to Do/ Buy for the Diet

Here are some things that you can buy for the diet to be a success.

Make lists

You can start by making a list of everything that you will need. Right from food to the other things, it is best for you to make a list and use it to buy the different things. You can make a hard copy and also a soft copy that you can carry with yourself when you go shopping.

Throw out foods

The next thing to do is to hit the kitchen and start assembling all the foods that are banned by the diet. Start with all the junk food and then move to the processed foods. Right from biscuits to cakes and other foods that are packaged need to be thrown out. You can then throw out any sauces and condiments, as they will contain sugar and other ingredients that contain carbs. You can either give it to your neighbor or donate to a soup kitchen.

Buy in bulk

Next, you should hit the supermarket and but the different things. You will have to prepare a list and go after each of the items. Those that aren't sure what to buy can do a simple internet search and find a ready list of items to buy for the low carb diet. It will work out to be cost effective if you buy the foods in bulk. You can buy it from a wholesaler and have him bring in the same foods on a monthly basis. You can also try ordering online, as that will save you time and effort.

Organize

The next step is to organize everything. You should place all the foods in your kitchen in a neat-stacked manner. This will allow you easy access to them and you can start cooking immediately. You should organize in such a way that the ingredients you need most are placed in the first row and you can easily reach them. Doing so will also encourage you to cook more often at home instead of ordering take away.

BMI

BMI refers to body mass index. You should calculate your BMI to check whether it is well within the range or off. Everybody has a certain range within which their BMI should lie and is based on their height and weight. There is a simple equation for it that you can use to calculate your BMI. But you can also use an online site where you type in the numbers and check your BMI. You can then check whether you lie within the right range.

Weighing machine

It is important for you to buy yourself a weighing machine. You should measure your weight from time to time to see if you have lost any substantial weight. The machine should be accurate. You can try buying a digital one as opposed to a mechanical one. You can weight yourself once every 2 weeks and then record it. You can try buying a machine that remembers your previous weights for you.

Tape

Apart from a weighing machine, you should also buy yourself a tape. You can measure your waist and check whether you have lost any inches. You should check and record it once at the very beginning of the journey and then keep measuring every now and then.

Body fat machine

You can also make use of a body fat machine. As you know, even a slim person might have a lot of fat in their bodies. So, it is important for you to measure your fat content from time to time and not limit it to measuring your weight alone. You can buy one online and that will help you measure the amount of fat that lies in your body. You can measure it from time to time. There is a set list that tells you the ideal amount of fat that should lie in a person's body. It differs from man to woman to child.

Utensils

The next step is for you to buy the utensils that you will be using to cook your low carb meals. You can buy yourself a slow cooker that will help cook your meals with ease and also maintain most of the nutrition in it. You can buy a pressure cooker that will cook food real fast. An instant pot will act as both and will also keep your food warm. You can buy a timer as well, which will help you keep track in the kitchen.

Gym equipment

As you know, you must exercise in order to lose your excess weight. Apart from coming up with an exercise plan, you should also buy yourself some gym equipment. These can be dumbbells, yoga mats etc. Buy yourself anything that will motivate you to start working out. It need not always be traditional equipment alone. You can try other things such as medicine ball, battle ropes etc. They will help you avail a good burn and you won't have to hit the gym.

These are some things that you can buy and do to start with the ketogenic diet.

Chapter 6:
Staying Put and Some Precautions to Observe

Here are some things that you should do in remaining put with the ketogenic diet.

Find a friend

The first thing to do is to find a friend that will support you. He or she can also act as a partner when you take up the diet. You will have company when you take up the different aspects of the diet. It need not always be a friend. You can ask a sibling, a colleague or even your spouse to join in. you will find it easy to prepare the food as well and will not have to prepare two or more meals at a time.

Make a group

You can also find and join a ketogenic group. They might meet up regularly to discuss the diet and you can do the same. You can find a group online and join in. But if there is no such group that meets then you can start one by yourself. Ask amongst your family members and friends if anyone is on the low carb diet and invite them over. You can then ask them to invite their friends and them theirs. Once you form the group, you can hold regular meetings and discuss the various aspects of the diet.

Reward yourself

It is important for any person to reward himself or herself from time to time in order to remain motivated. As you know, the cheat meal works best as a reward. You can follow the diet rigorously for a month and then treat yourself to a nice meal at your favorite restaurant. Some people prefer not to cheat and so, they can buy themselves something nice and memorable. Maybe a nice pair of shoes or a camera will cut it. However, try not to do it too often, as that will cause it to lose its value.

Profess about it

One good way to help the diet work better for you is by professing about it. This means that you speak about the diet with others and tell them how good it is. You can also speak about your own journey. The best way to tell many people about it is by making use of a blog or your social media. You can detail your experiences on the site and inform people about it. You can maintain a digital diary of it in order to tell people about your experience. But you have to prepare for feedback of all type. You might not always get positive comments and must be prepared to put up with negative comments that some people will post on purpose. You should learn to ignore it and focus on the positive comments.

Pregnant women

When it comes to taking precautions on the diet, pregnant women will have to exercise the most. You can speak with your doctor first and ask if it is fine for you to take up the ketogenic diet. She might tell you to do certain things while on the diet that will prove to be beneficial for your body. Even if you have been on the diet before getting pregnant then you must speak to the physician and ask for any supplements to be consumed.

New mothers

New mothers will require a lot of strength to recover from birthing and so; the low carb diet might not be an ideal one.

However, you must speak with your doctor about it and ask if you can take it up. Again, she might prescribe some supplements that you can consume to attain all the nutrients that are required by your body. She might also tell you the right time to start with the diet.

Children

If you as a parent are keen on getting your child started on the diet, then you should speak with their doctor first. Ask them if you can put them on the diet and also a meal plan to follow. That will make it easy for you to prepare the meals for your children. They might also need some supplements when on the diet and you should ask about the same. Exercise will be a must for children and so, you will have to encourage them to exercise regularly. They can take part in sports activities in school and avail the benefits.

Elders

Elders too must exercise some precaution when it comes to taking up the ketogenic diet. They should ask the doctor first and then take it up. Some might have to take supplements that will help them remain fit. They will also need a modified low carb diet based on their existing food habits and the amount of weight that they wish to lose.

Medications

Some people might have certain conditions such as diabetes and might consume medicines on a regular basis. Such people must speak with their doctor before taking up any diet. The doctor will be able to advise them correctly and tell them whether or not they can take up a certain diet. They might also be asked to follow a particular tailor made plan that will suit their bodies.

Supplements

It is a must for people to find out if a certain supplement will suit their body. Don't take something over the counter unless you are sure how it will work for you. You can ask your doctor first and then buy it. Apart from the vitamin supplements, you can also try some natural herbs and extracts, as they will further boost your body's capacity to lose weight and remain healthy and fit.

These form the different precautions that you have to observe while on the ketogenic low carb diet.

Chapter 7:
Recipes for Breakfast

Chocolate Raspberry Protein Shake
Ingredients

- 8 ounces almond milk (unsweetened)

- 2 ounces heavy cream

- 1 scoop Chocolate Whey Isolate Powder

- ½ tbsp. Sugar free raspberry syrup

- ½ cup crushed ice (you could add more or less as per your liking)

Method

1. Put all the ingredients in the blender and mix well. You have to ensure that the mixture is smooth.

Cucumber Pancakes
Ingredients

- 2 Cucumbers (shredded)

- 2 cups almond flour

- 3 eggs

- 2 tsp. dried basil

- 2 tsp. dried parsley

- Salt and Pepper to taste

- 3 tbsp. Butter

Instructions

1. Take a small mixing bowl and add the shredded cucumber, along with the basil and the almond flour.

2. Mix the ingredients well. Once the cucumber is coated well with the flour, add the parsley, pepper and the salt to the bowl.

3. Ensure that the taste of the mixture is well balanced.

4. You can make close to 10 patties from the mixture that you have just made.

5. Take a large non – stick sauce pan and place it on a medium flame.

6. Add one teaspoon to the pan. Once the butter has started warming up, add the patties and cook them one after the other.

7. Ensure that you remove the patty off the pan when it is brown on both sides.

White chocolate almond protein drink

Ingredients

- 8 ounces almond milk (unsweetened milk)

- ½ packet artificial sweetener

- 2 ounces heavy cream

- 1 scoop Vanilla Whey powder

- ½ tbsp. sugar free white chocolate syrup

- ½ cup crushed ice (you could add more or less as per your liking)

Method

1. Put all the ingredients in the blender and mix well. You have to ensure that the mixture is smooth.

Onion and Cheese Quiche

Ingredients

- 3 cups Colby jack cheese (divide the cups of cheese into two halves)

- 1tbsp. butter (a little more to grease the pan)

- ½ cup finely chopped white onion

- 6 large eggs (organic or free range)

- 1 cup heavy cream

- ½ tsp. salt

- ½ tsp. black pepper (ground)

- 1tsp. thyme (dried)

Method

1. You will first have to preheat the oven to 300 degrees Celsius.

2. Take a skillet and place it on medium flame. Once the skillet has warmed, add the butter to the pan and melt. Once the butter has melted, add the vegetables to the skillet and cook. Once the onions are soft and translucent, remove the skillet and cool the vegetables down.

3. Take a quiche pan and grease it well. Add one half of the shredded cheese to the bottom of the pan.

4. Add half the vegetables to the pan. Make a clean layer of the cheese.

5. Crack the eggs in a large bowl and mix well. Add the spices and the cream and continue to whisk. Mix it well enough so that the mixture is frothy.

6. Add the egg mixture to the quiche pan and distribute it evenly over the cheese and the vegetables.

7. Bake the quiche for thirty minutes and pull the quiche out when it has set well and is lightly puffy and golden in the center.

8. Cut the quiche and refrigerate it. You can have the quiche thrice a week for breakfast.

Baked Bacon and Eggs

Ingredients

- 4 tbsp. butter

- 6 large eggs

- 1 ½ cup cheddar cheese (grated)

- 1 ½ heavy cream (heat it till it is lukewarm)

- 12 slices bacon (cooked and crumbled)

- Salt and pepper

Method

1. You will first need to preheat the oven to 300 degrees Fahrenheit.

2. Take six glass ramekins – preferably 6 ounces in size and grease them well with butter.

3. Crack the six eggs into each of the ramekins.

4. Cover the eggs with the cheese and the cream, a neat layer, and add salt and pepper to taste.

5. Place the ramekins in a large pan and fill the pan up with water to cover half the ramekins. It is best to do it this way since you will not be able to place the ramekins

in the pan correctly if you have filled the pan up with water.

6. Place the pan in the oven and let the eggs bake for twenty minutes. You will need to ensure that the cheese has completely melted and the egg whites are almost cooked.

7. Crumble two slices of the bacon over each ramekin and serve it hot. If you are making it just for one person or two people, you could change the proportions of the ingredients.

Cheddar Garlic Biscuits

Ingredients

- 5 cups almond flour

- 12 ounces Colby jack cheese (shredded)

- 10 tbsp. butter

- 16 ounces cream cheese

- 4 large eggs or 6 medium eggs

- 4 tsp. garlic (granulated)

- 2 tsp. baking soda

- 2 tsp. Xanthan gum

- 2 tsp. sea salt

Method

1. Take a cookie sheet and grease it well. Line it with parchment paper if you do not want to grease it.

2. Then preheat the oven to300 degrees Fahrenheit.

3. Process the shredded cheese and one cup of the almond flour in a food processor till they have blended well and are granular. Keep this aside.

4. Take a large mixing bowl. Add the butter and the cream cheese to the bowl and place. You have to melt the better a little. Once it has melted, mix the butter and the cheese together. Make sure that the mixture is smooth and glossy.

5. Add the eggs to the mixture and continue to whisk. Make sure that the mixture is smooth and glossy.

6. Add the garlic, the Xanthan gum, baking soda and the salt to the mixture.

7. Add the remaining almond flour and cheese mixture to the egg mixture and whisk well.

8. Once the ingredients have blended well, add the almond flour that is left and continue to fold the mixture well. You have to ensure that the dough has formed.

9. Take a tablespoon and scoop the dough and place it on the cookie sheet. Keep the cookies one inch apart. If you want you could flatten the dough a little to ensure that you have a smooth biscuit.

10. Place the cookie sheet in the oven and bake for thirty minutes. You will need to leave the biscuits in till they have a golden brown color.

11. Remove the biscuits from the oven and cool to room temperature. You can serve it with a glass of milk.

Bacon and Eggs

Ingredients

- 2 tbsp. butter

- 16 slices bacon (has to be meaty)

- 2 carrots

- 5 Broccoli florets

- 6 Celery sticks

- White onion

- 5 large eggs

- 1 cup Colby jack cheese (shredded)

Method

1. Peel and cut the carrots into thin slices.

2. Chop all the other vegetables finely.

3. Cut the bacon into thin slices or strips.

4. Take a skillet and place it on a medium flame. Add the butter to the skillet. Once it has melted, add the bacon and the vegetables to the skillet.

5. Stir the vegetables and the bacon well. You will need to cook the bacon and the vegetables till the bacon turns crispy around the edges and the vegetables are caramelized well.

6. Make sure that the mixture has spread evenly in the skillet. You could then make five small holes in the middle of the layer.

7. Crack the eggs into the small holes. You will need to continue to cook the vegetables and the eggs in the skillet. You could cover the skillet with a lid. This will help in cooking the eggs well. If you prefer having a liquid yolk, you could cook the eggs without the lid.

8. When the eggs have been cooked well, you could spread the cheese over the top and let the cheese melt on the medium flame. Serve the bacon and eggs hot!

Pumpkin Pancakes

Ingredients

- 2 pumpkins (shredded)

- 2 cups almond flour

- 3 eggs

- 2 tsp. dried basil

- 2 tsp. dried parsley

- Salt and Pepper to taste

- 3 tbsp. Butter

Instructions

1. Take a small mixing bowl and add the pumpkin, along with the basil and the almond flour.

2. Mix the ingredients well. Once the pumpkin is coated well with the flour, add the parsley, pepper and the salt to the bowl.

3. Ensure that the taste of the mixture is well balanced.

4. You can make close to 10 patties from the mixture that you have just made.

5. Take a large non – stick sauce pan and place it on a medium flame.

6. Add one teaspoon to the pan. Once the butter has started warming up, add the patties and cook them one after the other.

7. Ensure that you remove the patty off the pan when it is brown on both sides.

Simple crepes

Ingredients

- 1 cup almond flour

- 2 eggs, beaten

- ½ cup almond milk

- 1 tablespoon grass fed butter

- 2 teaspoons vanilla extract

- 1 cup sugar free chocolate chips

- 3 small ripe bananas

Method

1. Start by mashing the bananas.

2. Add it to a bowl along with the butter, milk, and vanilla extract and mix until well combined.

3. Add in the beaten eggs and the flour and mix into a batter.

4. You can add in water to thin the batter.

5. Heat a griddle and pour 1 ladle of the batter on it at a time.

6. Once it browns on one side, flip it over and brown it on the other side.

7. Serve hot with some banana slices on top.

Avocado omelets

Ingredients

- 1 ripe avocado

- 1 red onion, chopped

- 1 tomato, chopped

- 1 tablespoon oil

- 3 eggs, beaten

- Salt to taste

- Pepper to taste

Method

1. Start by removing the seed from the avocado and scoop out the flesh.

2. Add it to a bowl along with the chopped onion, tomato, salt and pepper and mix until well combined.

3. Add in the eggs and beat well.

4. Heat a pan and ladle the batter on it to form omelets.

5. Serve hot.

Asparagus with Parmesan

Ingredients

- 10 asparagus stems

- 1 tablespoon grass fed butter

- 4 cloves garlic, chopped

- Salt to taste

- Chili flakes to taste

- ½ cup parmesan cheese

Method

1. Start by cutting the asparagus stems in half and add to boiling water to soften.

2. Meanwhile, add the butter, garlic, salt and chili to a pan and melt.

3. Fish out the asparagus and add it to the butter mix and toss.

4. Sprinkle the cheese on top and serve with the cheese melting on top.

Coconut pancakes

Ingredients

- 1 cup almond flour

- 1 cup coconut flakes or desiccated coconut

- 1 cup coconut milk, or more as needed

- Salt to taste

- Chili flakes to taste

Method

1. Start by adding the coconut milk, salt and chili to a bowl.

2. Add in the flour, coconut flakes and mix until well combined.

3. You can add in some water at this point to make the batter more pliable.

4. Heat a griddle and add in a ladleful of the batter and wait for it to cook on one side before flipping it over and browning the other side.

5. Serve hot.

Spicy devilled eggs

Ingredients

- 4 hardboiled eggs

- 2 jalapeño peppers, chopped

- Salt to taste

- Mustard to taste

- 1 lemon, juiced

- Coriander leaves to sprinkle

Method

1. Start by cutting the eggs into half diagonally.

2. Remove the yellow core and add to a bowl.

3. Add in the salt and pepper along with the chopped jalapeños and give it a good mix.

4. Add in the mustard and lemon juice.

5. Spoon the yellow back into the centers of the eggs, sprinkle with the coriander leaves and serve.

Peanut butter pancakes

Ingredients

- 2 cups almond flour
- 2 cups almond milk
- 3 eggs
- 1 tablespoon grass fed butter
- 1 cup peanut butter
- 2 tablespoons sweetener

Method

1. Start by adding the eggs, butter and milk to a bowl and give it a good mix.
2. Add in the sweetener and peanut butter and mix well.
3. Add in the flour and make a smooth batter.
4. Heat a griddle and use a ladle to pour the batter on it.
5. Allow it to brown on one side and then flip to brown on the other side.
6. Serve it with some peanut butter.

Sautéed cabbage

Ingredients

- 1 small cabbage

- 2 tablespoons grass fed butter

- Salt to taste

- Pepper to taste

Method

1. Start by separating the leaves of the cabbage and wash it.

2. Chop the leaves into small slices.

3. Add the butter to a pan and add in the cabbage.

4. Allow it to brown and soften.

5. Add in the salt and pepper and serve hot.

Salmon with pineapple

Ingredients

- 1 salmon fillet

- 4 slices pineapple

- 2 small onions

- 2 tablespoons rosemary leaves

- Salt to taste

- Pepper to taste

- Mint to sprinkle

- Olive oil to drizzle

Method

1. Preheat the oven at 350 degrees Fahrenheit.

2. Start by place the salmon fillet in a bowl.

3. Drizzle the oil over it and sprinkle the salt and pepper on top.

4. Rub it in.

5. Sprinkle the rosemary over it.

6. Now place the onions over a tray in a straight line.

7. Place the salmon fillet over it.

8. Now place the pineapple slices over it.

9. Bake the salmon for 15 to 20 minutes or until the fish is cooked.

10. Serve hot.

Chapter 8:
Recipes for Salads

Chicken, Tomato and Bacon Salad
Ingredients

For the Salad

- 2 large uncooked chicken breasts (cut them into chunks that are one inch each)

- 4 tsp. Canadian Steak Brand (you could use any brand that you want)

- 4 tbsp. butter

- 10 slices bacon

- 2 small tomatoes

- 3 ounces Muenster cheese

For the dressing

- 3 tbsp. butter

- 2 raw eggs (preferably eggs from a pastured chicken. This egg will be richer)

- 3 ounces mayonnaise

- 3 tsp. lemon juice

- 1 tsp. salt

Method

The Salad

1. Add the Canadian steak seasoning to the chicken and spread it neatly.

2. Take a pan and place it on a medium flame and add the butter. When the butter begins to melt, add the chicken breasts and sauté it. Make sure that it is cooked through before you remove it off the pan. Leave it aside to cool down to room temperature.

3. Cut the bacon into thin strips. Sauté the strips in a pan on a medium flame until they are crispy. Drain the fat from the pan. Leave the bacon strips on paper towels to drain all the oil.

The Dressing

1. Take a small pan and add the butter to it. Place the pan on low heat. Once the butter melts pull the pan off the flame and leave the butter to cool.

2. Add the yolk to the butter and whisk the two well till the mixture has become glossy and smooth.

3. Add the remaining ingredients and whisk till the mixture is smooth.

The finished Salad

1. Take a plate and add all the ingredients and the dressing and mix them well.

2. Ensure that the ingredients are coated well with the dressing.

Apple and Spinach Salad

Ingredients

- 2 cups spinach leaves (preferably baby spinach leaves. Ensure that they are washed well.)

- 1 cup red onion (sliced fine)

- 5 tbsp. blue cheese (crumbled)

- 1 apple (cut it into small cubes)

Method

1. Take a small bowl.

2. Add the apple cubes to the bowl.

3. Add the spinach to the bowl. Lay the onions on the spinach.

4. You could add your very own choice of dressing.

Creamy Chicken Salad

Ingredients

For the Salad

- 1-cup chicken (cooked and diced. Ensure that the meat is darker since that makes it tastier)

- ¼ cup celery (diced finely)

- ¼ cup green onion (sliced)

For the dressing

- 2 ounces cream cheese (softened)

- 2 ounces mayonnaise

- ½ tsp. tarragon (dried)

- ¼ tsp. thyme (dried)

- Salt and pepper to taste

Method

1. Take a mixing bowl and add the cream cheese and the mayonnaise. Whisk the two till the mixture is smooth.

2. Add the spices to the cream cheese mixture and whisk well.

3. Take a large salad bowl and add the chicken, celery and the green onions.

4. Coat the ingredients with the dressing.

5. You could eat the salad in a lettuce leaf or eat it out of the bowl.

Egg Salad

Ingredients

- 6 large eggs

- ¼ cup mayonnaise

- 1 tbsp. melted butter

- ¼ tsp. mustard (preferably ground)

- 1/6 cup white onion (minced finely)

- Salt and pepper to taste

Method

1. Take a large pot and fill it with cold water. Leave the eggs in the pot and boil them. Cook them for ten minutes.

2. Remove the pot from the heat and remove as much water as you can from the pot. Leave the eggs in the pot and add cold water to the pot.

3. Let the eggs sit in the water for a few minutes.

4. Remove the eggs from the pot and pat them dry. Peel the eggs off and make sure that the shell is not found on the egg.

5. Take a large mixing bowl and chop the eggs into slices. You could either chop them into slices or cut them into small pieces of uniform size. Make sure that they all look the same. Do not mince the egg.

6. Add the other ingredients to the mixing bowl and mix them well. Leave the salad in the refrigerator and serve cold.

Mashed Avocado salad

Ingredients

- 2 ripe avocados

- 1 big tomato

- 1 red onion

- 1 slit green chili

- 1 large lemon

- Salt to taste

- Fresh parsley leaves

Method

1. Start by using a sharp knife to cut the avocado in half. Now use the same to remove the seed from the center.

2. Use a spoon to scoop out the insides of the avocado and add it to a bowl.

3. Chop the onion and tomatoes into small bite sized piece.

4. Add it to the avocado mash and give it a good mix.

5. Add in the chili and salt and mix everything until well combined.

6. Sprinkle the parsley leaves on top and serve the salad as is or refrigerate for an hour and serve cold.

Bean salad

Ingredients

- 1 cup red beans

- 1 cup cannellini beans

- 1 cup chickpeas

- 1 cup mung beans

- 2 tomatoes

- 1 onion

- 1 zucchini

- 1 lemon

- 1 tablespoon olive oil

- Salt to taste

- Pepper to taste

- Parsley to sprinkle

Method

1. Start by soaking all the beans in water overnight and then boiling them for 45 minutes or use them out of a can after washing them thoroughly.

2. Add them to a bowl and toss them around.

3. In a small bowl add the olive oil, lemon juice, salt and pepper and mix everything well.

4. Chop the onion, tomatoes and zucchini into bean sized pieces and add to the bowl.

5. Add the dressing to the salad and give it a good mix. Everything should combine well.

6. Sprinkle the parsley on top and serve warm.

Spinach soup

Ingredients

- 2 bunches fresh spinach

- 4 spring onion sprigs

- 2 cups water

- 2 tablespoons olive oil

- Salt to taste

- 2 tablespoons almond flour

- 2 tablespoons warm water

Method

1. Start by separating the spinach leaves individually and wash them. You can keep the stocks for this soup.

2. Cut the bulbs of the spring onions into small pieces.

3. Add the oil to a pan and let it heat.

4. Add the chopped onion bulbs and sauté it.

5. Once done, tear up the spinach and spring onion leaves and allow them to wilt.

6. Once done, add everything to a liquidizer along with the water and create a smooth paste.

7. Add it back to the pan and toss in the salt and pepper.

8. Add the almond flour to a small bowl along with the warm water and make a smooth paste.

9. Add the paste to the soup and allow it to thicken.

10. Once it is thick enough, switch off the heat and serves the soup hot.

Mixed fruit salad

Ingredients

- 1 orange

- 1 apple

- 1 red onion

- 1 tablespoon olive oil

- 1 tablespoon honey

- Salt to taste

- Pepper to taste

- 2 tablespoons walnuts, chopped

Method

1. Start by cutting the orange and apples into small pieces.

2. Cut the onions into rings.

3. Add the oil to a pan and add the onion rings to sauté until they turn translucent.

4. Add the fruits to a bowl along with the onions.

5. Drizzle the honey over it and give it a good mix.

6. Add in the salt and pepper and also the chopped walnuts and serve.

Banana salad

Ingredients

- 2 large bananas

- 1 cup pomegranate seeds

- 1 cup grass fed yogurt

- 1 teaspoon honey

- A pinch of salt

- Mint leaves to sprinkle

Method

1. Start by adding the bananas to a bowl and use a masher to mash it.

2. Add in the pomegranate seeds and set it aside.

3. Now add the honey and salt to the yogurt and give it a good mix.

4. Add it to the banana mash and give it a good mix.

5. Sprinkle the mint leaves and serve.

Chicken and basil soup

Ingredients

-   2 chicken breasts

-   ½ cup fresh basil leaves

-   1 cup chicken stock

-   Salt to taste

-   Pepper to taste

-   1 red chili

-   Parsley to sprinkle

Method

1. Start by adding the stock to a pan and switch on the heat.

2. Add in the chicken breasts and poach it until the meat is tender.

3. Don't overcook it.

4. Once done, remove the breasts out and add in chopped basil to the stock.

5. Add in the salt and pepper and mix it.

6. Use a fork to shred the chicken breasts.

7. Add it to a bowl and ladle the clear soup over it.

8. You can add in some more pepper to enhance its taste.

Leafy salad

Ingredients

- 1/2 cup lettuce leaves

- ½ cup rocket leaves

- ½ cup arugula leaves

- ½ cup bok choy

- ½ cup spinach leaves

- 1 tablespoon olive oil

- 2 tablespoons roasted pine nuts

- 1 tablespoon roasted white sesame seeds

- Salt to taste

- Pepper to taste

Method

1. Start by boiling water in a pan.

2. Once it boils add in the spinach leaves and bok choy and get them to wilt.

3. Once it does, fish them out and add to a bowl.

4. Chop the rest of the leaves into bite sized bits and add to the spinach.

5. In a small bowl add in the olive oil, salt, pepper and mix well.

6. Drizzle it over the salad and mix until well combined.

7. Sprinkle toasted pine nuts and sesame seeds and serve.

Tomato Rasam

Ingredients

- 3 tomatoes, chopped

- 2 cups water

- 1 teaspoon cumin seeds

- 1 teaspoon black pepper corns

- 1 teaspoon fenugreek seeds

- 2 dried red chilies

- 1 teaspoon olive oil

- 1 teaspoon mustard seeds

- Salt to taste

- Coriander leaves

Method

1. Start by adding the cumin seeds, black pepper corns, fenugreek seeds and red chilies to a small pan and allow them to heat up.

2. Add them to a coffee grinder and make a fine powder.

3. Add the oil to a pan and add in the mustard seeds.

4. Once they splutter, add in the fine powder.

5. Add in the chopped tomatoes along with the water and allow it to cook.

6. Serve hot with a sprinkling of fresh coriander leaves on top.

Dal soup

Ingredients

- 1 cup yellow lentil

- 1 teaspoon turmeric powder

- 1 teaspoon oil

- 1 teaspoon mustard

- 1 green chili slit

- Salt to taste

- Coriander to sprinkle

Method

1. Add the lentil to boiling water and cook for 40 minutes or until soft.

2. Once done, use the back of your ladle to mash the lentil into a puree.

3. In a small pan, add in the oil and mustard and allow it to splutter.

4. Add it to the soup along with the chili and salt and mix.

5. Cover and cook for 5 minutes.

6. Serve with sprinkled coriander on top.

Chapter 9:
Recipes for Mains

Spinach, bacon and shallots

Ingredients

- 8 ounces raw spinach

- ¼ cup white onion (chopped)

- ¼ cup shallots (chopped)

- ¼ pound raw slices of bacon

- 1 tbsp. butter

Method

1. Slice the strips of bacon into thinner pieces.

2. Take a skillet and add butter to it.

3. Add the onions, bacon and the shallots to the skillet. Sauté for twenty minutes. Once the onions have turned translucent and the bacon has cooked, add the spinach leaves to the skillet.

4. Sauté the leaves on a medium flame. Keep stirring and make sure that you turn the leaves over so that they are cooked well. This would also mix the bacon and the onion together.

5. Keep stirring till the spinach has wilted. Serve hot.

Kale with bacon, onion and garlic

Ingredients

- 2 large bunches of kale leaves

- 2 cups chopped onions

- 4 cloves garlic

- 6 slices raw bacon

- 4 tbsp. butter

Method

1. Take a skillet and place it on a medium flame and add butter to it.

2. Cut the bacon into small strips or pieces and add them to the skillet.

3. Cook the bacon well.

4. Add the onion to the skillet and sauté till it is translucent. Add the garlic to the skillet.

5. Once the garlic and the onions have cooked, add the kale leaves.

6. Sauté on a medium flame and stir occasionally. You have to ensure that you are turning the leaves over to cook them well. This will mix the onion and the bacon well.

7. Cook the kale till it is softened. This may take an hour.

Decadent Keto Meatloaf Recipe

Ingredients

- 8 tsp. Dijon mustard

- 8 tbsp. butter for sautéing

- 2 cups almond flour

- 4 tbsp. thyme leaves*

- 1 cup minced fresh parsley leaves*

- 2 cups shredded (not dry grated) Parmesan cheese

- 8 T Ellen's Low Carb Barbecue sauce

- 1 cup heavy cream

- 8 large eggs

- 4 tbsp. fresh basil leaves, chopped fine*

- 24 ounces of cream cheese, softened to room temp

- 8 cups shredded cheddar cheese, minced in food processor.

- 4 cups chopped green pepper

- 4 tsp. salt

- ½ tsp. unflavored gelatin

- 8 pounds 85% ground beef

- 4 pound Italian sausage

- 2 tsp. ground black pepper

- 24 ounces chopped white onion (measure by weight)

- 16 garlic cloves, minced

Procedure

1. You will need to preheat the oven to 300 degrees Celsius.

2. Take a 12 x 20 glass-baking dish and grease it well with butter.

3. Take a small bowl and add the almond flour and the Parmesan cheese to it. You will need to mix it well together.

4. In another bowl, add the cheddar cheese and the softened cheese together. You will need to stir well to ensure that the mixture is smooth without any lumps. You will have to be able to spread it over bread without any lumps.

5. Take a saucepan and place it over a medium flame. When the pan is hot, add the oil to the pan. Once the oil has warmed, add the garlic, onion and the pepper to the pan. You will need to cook the ingredients till the onions have turned translucent and soft. This will generally take ten minutes.

6. Remove the saucepan off the flame and leave the ingredients to cool.

7. Once the onions and the garlic have cooled, add them to a food processor and mince them. You will need to ensure that it has great consistency.

8. Take another small bowl and whisk the eggs in the bowl. You need to ensure that there are no bubbles in the bowl. Add the spices to the egg mixture along with the salt, pepper and the barbecue sauce. Once the ingredients have mixed well, add the cream to the bowl and mix.

9. Sprinkle the gelatin onto the mixture and leave it to set for ten minutes.

10. Chop the Italian sausage and the beef finely. Place them on a cutting board and mix them well. You need to ensure that the mixture is fine and you cannot differentiate too much between the sausage and the beef with the flour. You have to ensure that the mixture does not stick too much. If you find that it does, you will need to add the Parmesan cheese to it one spoon at a time!

11. Continue to knead the mixture for a while. Make sure that it is soft. If it starts to get tough, stop kneading it immediately.

12. Add the meatloaf mixture to the egg mixture and stir well. You will have to mix all the other ingredients to this very mixture. You could add once ingredient at a time and mix well to ensure that the taste has evenly spread throughout the mixture.

13. Add the flour one spoon at a time to the mixture and continue to stir. You will need to stop when the ingredients have blended well together.

14. Take a cookie sheet and cover it with wax paper or grease it well with butter or oil. Place the mixture meat on the sheet. Once the meat has sat well, add the mixture of the cream and the cheese to the meat. Cover the layer of meat well.

15. Start to roll the wax paper from one end with the meat. You will need to remove the paper off the sheet.

16. You will need to seal the ends of the roll to ensure that the cheese and the cream do not ooze out.

17. Take a baking tray and grease it well. Place the roll on the tray and bake it in the oven.

18. You will need to ensure that the meat is cooked well. You can check whether it is cooked well by using a thermometer. The meat has to be 150 degrees Celsius.

19. Place the roll in the baking tray and bake in the oven. It will take a minimum of five or ten minutes to cook the meat. You could leave it in longer to ensure that it is cooked well from every end.

20. Serve the loaf with sauce!

Herb Baked Salmon

Ingredients

- 1 pound salmon fillets
- 2 ounces sesame oil
- ¼ cup tamari soy sauce
- ½ tsp. garlic (minced)
- ¼ tsp. ginger (ground)
- ¼ tsp. basil
- ½ tsp. oregano leaves
- ¼ tsp. thyme
- ¼ tsp. rosemary
- ¼ tsp. tarragon
- 2 ounces butter
- ¼ cup fresh mushrooms (chopped)
- ¼ cup green onions (chopped)

Method

1. Cut the salmon fillets to fill one cup.
2. Take a small plastic bag and place the salmon in the bag. Leave it in the deep freeze.
3. Mix the sauce, the oil and the spices together.

4. Add this mixture to the salmon and place the salmon back into the refrigerator. Leave it to marinate for a few hours.

5. Preheat the oven to 300 degrees Fahrenheit.

6. Take a baking tray and line it with foil.

7. Take the salmon out of the deep freeze and place it in the pan. Make sure that the salmon is all in one layer.

8. Bake the salmon fillets for 15 – 20 minutes.

9. While the salmon is baking, you will need to start cooking the vegetables.

10. Take a small bowl and add the vegetables to it. Melt the butter and add the butter to the bowl. Make sure that all the vegetables are coated well with the butter.

11. Remove the pan from the oven and add the butter and vegetable mixture to the pan.

12. Leave the pan back in the oven for fifteen minutes. Serve it hot!

Baked Salmon

Ingredients

- 4 cloves garlic

- 12 tbsp. olive oil (light)

- 2 tsp. basil (dried)

- 2 tsp. salt

- 2 tsp. black pepper (ground)

- 2 tbsp. lemon juice

- 2 tbsp. fresh parsley (chopped)

- 12 ounces salmon fillets

Method

1. Preheat the oven 375 degree Fahrenheit.

2. Take a medium sized bowl and add the garlic, olive oil, salt, basil and the pepper and mix well. Make sure that the taste has spread evenly throughout the mixture. Add the lemon juice and the parsley to the mixture.

3. Take a baking dish and add the salmon fillets. Cover the fillets with the marinade and leave them for an hour. Turn the fillets over.

4. Place the salmon in an aluminum foil and seal the salmon in it.

5. Place the salmon in a baking dish and leave it in the oven for fifty minutes to cook.

6. Serve hot.

Chicken Guadalajara

Ingredients

- 4 tbsp. butter

- 8 ounces white onions (chopped finely)

- 6 garlics (minced cloves)

- 8 boneless, skinless, chicken breast halves

- 6 ounces cans diced tomatoes

- 6 ounces cans of green chilies

- 1 cup whipped cream

- 1 cup chicken broth

- 1 tsp. cayenne pepper

- 1 tsp. cumin (dried)

- 1 tsp. garlic powder

- 2 tsp. sea salt

- Grated cheddar cheese (garnish)

- Sour cream (garnish)

- Salsa (garnish)

Method

1. Wash the chicken breasts and pat them dry. Cut them into slices.

2. Take a medium sized skillet and place it on a medium flame. Melt the butter in the skillet and add the onions and garlic to the skillet. Cook them till the onions are soft.

3. Add the chicken to the skillet and cook it well. Drain out all the fat from the chicken.

4. Reduce the heat and add the tomatoes and the chili to the skillet.

5. Cover the skillet and continue to cook it for another fifteen minutes.

6. Add the cream cheese to the skillet and stir till the cheese has melted well. Add the sour cream and mix well.

7. You will have to ensure that the chicken and the vegetables were coated well with cheese.

8. Add the broth to the sauce and mix well.

9. Top with garnishes and serve hot.

Pizza with Sausages

Ingredients

- 2 tbsp. olive oil

- 1 cauliflower head (trim and then chop the head into smaller pieces)

- 1 ounce white onion (minced)

- 3 tbsp. butter

- ½ cup water

- 4 eggs (2 large eggs)

- 3 cups mozzarella cheese (shredded and chopped into smaller pieces)

- 2 tsp. fennel seeds

- 3 tsp. Italian seasoning

- ½ cup parmesan (grated)

- 5 ounces Pizza Sauce (pick a sauce that is very low in carbohydrates)

- 1 pound Italian sausage (look for the sausage that has a very low amount of carbohydrates)

- 1 cup Italian cheese (preferably get the five cheese blend. You will have to shred the cheese.)

Method

For the crust

1. Preheat the oven to 400 degrees Fahrenheit.

2. Take a cookie sheet and grease it well with the olive oil.

3. Take a large skillet and place it on a medium flame.

4. Add the butter to the skillet and add the onions to the skillet and sauté them till they are translucent. Add the cauliflower to the skillet and cook it till it is almost done.

5. Add water to the skillet and cover the skillet. Leave the vegetables in till the cauliflower is cooked and soft.

6. Transfer the vegetables to a glass bowl and leave them to cool.

7. As the cauliflower is cooling, you will need to cook the Italian sausages. You will need to break them into smaller pieces and cook them well. Drain all the fat out from the skillet. Pat the sausages dry on a tissue paper to remove any excess fat. Leave these aside to cool.

8. Once the cauliflower has cooled down, take three cups of the cauliflower and place it in a food processor or a blender. You will need to blend it till the cauliflower has turned into a smooth puree. Move the puree into a mixing bowl.

9. Add the eggs to the mixing bowl along with the cheese and the spices. Blend them well. Now add the Parmesan cheese and mix it well!

10. Add the cauliflower puree to the cookie sheet and spread it neatly with a spatula. You will have to have a certain thickness all around the sheet.

11. Bake the crust in the oven for twenty minutes. Remove the crust when you find that it has turned brown at the edges.

12. While the pizza crust is in the oven, you will need to chop the sausages into fine pieces. You could either cut the sausage or process it in the food processor.

13. Pour the pizza sauce in a saucepan and add the Italian sausage to the pan.

14. Cook the sausage in the pizza sauce till the sauce has become thick.

For the pizza

1. Once the crust is cooked, you can remove it from the oven and turn the oven settings to boil. Leave the oven shelf four inches from the broiler.

2. Pour the sausage and sauce mixture over the crust. Spread the mixture over the crust using a spatula. You will have a thin coating of the sauce and the sausage. You could add more sausage and sauce to the crust if you want.

3. Leave the pizza in the oven and broil it till the cheese melts. You have to ensure that the cheese has begun to bubble.

4. Remove the pizza from the oven and cut how many ever slices you want.

Roast pork

Ingredients

- 3 pounds boneless pork shoulder
- 1 tablespoon caraway seed
- 2 teaspoons marjoram, dried
- Salt to taste
- Pepper to taste
- 1 tablespoon olive oil
- ½ cup water
- 2 tablespoons white wine vinegar
- 7 to 8 ounce sour cream

Method

1. Start by mixing the marjoram, salt, pepper and caraway seeds and sprinkle it all over the pork.

2. Use your hands to rub the mix all over the pork.

3. You can use a slow cooker for this dish.

4. Add the oil to the slow cooker and add the oil to it.

5. Once it heats, add the pork roast and turn it around on all sides to turn it brown.

6. Once it does, remove it out.

7. Add in the water, vinegar and cream to the pan and mix it until well combined.

8. Now add in the pork shoulder to it and close the slow cooker.

9. Pick the highest time setting on the slow cooker.

10. Once done, the meat should fall off the bone.

11. Serve it hot.

Simple beef stew

Ingredients

- 2 lbs. beef

- 5 cups beef broth

- Salt to taste

- Pepper to taste

- 1 teaspoon chili powder

- 1 teaspoon Worcestershire sauce

- 2 tablespoons olive oil

- 1 red onion, chopped

- 2 tablespoon garlic, chopped

- 3 medium carrots

- 4 medium celery sticks

Method

1. Start by add in the beef to a bowl and add the salt, pepper and chili powder to it.

2. Mix it until well combined.

3. Add the Worcestershire sauce to it and mix.

4. Set it aside.

5. Meanwhile, add the oil to a pan and allow it to heat.

6. Add in the garlic and brown it.

7. Add the onion, carrots and celery sticks.

8. Add the beef stock and allow it to come to a boil.

9. Add in the beef and wait for it to boil.

10. Cover with a lid and simmer it.

11. You must cook it for 1 to 2 hours or until the meat is completely cooked.

Shrimp with lemons

Ingredients

- 2 lbs. raw shrimp, deveined

- ¼ cup butter, cubed

- 1/4 cup fresh parsley leaves

- Salt to taste

- Pepper to taste

- 4 cloves garlic, chopped

- 1 lemon, juiced

- Parsley to sprinkle

Method

1. Preheat the oven to 375 degrees Fahrenheit.

2. Start by adding the butter, parsley, and garlic to a blender and whizz until everything combines well.

3. Add in the shrimps to it along with the salt and pepper and mix it.

4. Place shrimps on a baking tray and squeeze the lemon over it.

5. Place the tray in the oven and bake it for 15 minutes or until the shrimps are done.

6. Serve hot with a sprinkling of parsley leaves on top.

Tuna curry

Ingredients

- 1 cup tuna, chopped

- 1/2 cup walnuts, chopped

- 1/4 cup almonds, chopped

- 2 hardboiled eggs

- 2 tablespoons low carb mayo

- Salt to taste

- Chili powder to taste

- 1 tablespoon curry powder

- Parsley to sprinkle

Method

1. Start by adding the oil to a pan and add in the walnuts and almonds.

2. Once it browns, add the curry powder, salt and chili powder and give it a good mix.

3. Once it browns, add in the chopped tuna.

4. Add in enough water and cover it.

5. Once it cooks, ladle it into a bowl.

6. Place the boiled eggs on top and spoon over it some of the mayo.

7. Serve hot with cauliflower rice.

Mixed vegetable stir fry

Ingredients

- 2 tablespoons olive oil

- 1 cup mushrooms, chopped

- 1 red pepper, cut into matchsticks

- 4 spring onions, cut into matchsticks

- 1 cup red pumpkin, cut into matchsticks

- 1 tablespoon curry powder

- 1 tablespoon toasted coconut flakes

- Parsley leaves to sprinkle

Method

1. Start by adding the oil to a pan and toss in the onion.

2. Once its browns toss in the mushrooms, red pepper and pumpkin and brown them.

3. Add in the curry powder, coconut flakes and chili powder and sauté everything.

4. Add it to a bowl top with parsley and serve.

Stuffed tomatoes

Ingredients

- 6 large round tomatoes

- 2 tablespoons olive oil

- ½ cup chickpeas

- 1 large onion

- 1 lemon

- Salt to taste

- Chili powder to taste

- Parmesan cheese to sprinkle

Method

1. Preheat the oven to 350 degrees Fahrenheit.

2. Start by taking off ½ an inch from top of the tomatoes but don't discard them.

3. Use a spoon to remove the core and seeds of each tomato to create a cavity.

4. Add the chickpeas, chopped onion, lemon juice, chili powder and salt to it and mix until well combined.

5. Now use a tablespoon to add the mix into the tomatoes.

6. Cover the tomatoes with their tops and place them on a greased oven tray.

7. Sprinkle the cheese on top.

8. Bake them for 15 to 20 minutes or until the skin of the tomatoes are all wrinkled up.

9. Serve hot.

Cauliflower rice

Ingredients

- 1 cauliflower head

- 1 teaspoon oil

- 1 teaspoon cumin seeds

- ½ teaspoon turmeric powder

- Salt to taste

- Pepper to taste

Method

1. Start by separating the florets of the cauliflower.

2. Prepare a steamer.

3. Place the cauliflower in the steam basked and steam it until it cooks.

4. Meanwhile, add the oil to a pan along with the cumin seeds, turmeric, salt and pepper.

5. Add the florets to a grinder and grind to a coarse powder.

6. Add it to the mix and give it a good stir.

7. Serve hot.

Chapter 10:
Recipes for Snacks and Drinks

Keto Italian Meatballs
Ingredients

- 4 ounces minced white onion

- 2 tsp. Italian seasoning

  o tsp. sea salt

- 1 tsp. freshly ground black pepper

- 1 cup shredded Romano / parmesan /asiago mix

- 1 large eggs

- 1 pound ground beef (92% lean)

- 1 cup cold whole milk ricotta cheese

- 1 tbsp. olive oil

  o tsp. granulated garlic

Method

1. First preheat the oven to 350 degree Celsius.

2. Take a saucepan and place it on medium flame. Add the olive to the pan. Once the oil has heated, add the onions and sauté till they are translucent.

3. Once the onions have turned translucent, take the pan off the flame and leave the onions to cool.

4. Mince the Romano/ parmesan/ asiago mix in a blender or a food processor.

5. Take a large mixing bowl and add the eggs and the ricotta cheese to the bowl and mix well! Make sure that there are no lumps in the mixture and that it is smooth.

6. Add the salt, pepper and the remaining spices to the mixture and stir well. Ensure that the spices and the egg mixture have blended well.

7. Add the sautéed onions to the egg mixture along with the minced Romano / Parmesan / asiago mix. Add the ingredients well.

8. Add vinegar to the bowl and ensure that the mixture is smooth.

9. When the mixture has blended well, add the beef to the mixture. You will need to ensure that the mixture is well balanced once you add the beef to the mixture. Ensure that the taste is balanced throughout the mixture!

10. Divide the entire mixture in portions with one ounce each. You will have 20 sized pieces of the beef.

11. You will need to make a ball out of the 20 pieces that you make.

12. Grease a cookie sheet well with the olive oil and place the beef meatballs on the tray. Place the tray in the oven for twenty minutes! Make sure that they are brown on the outside before you serve them!

Crab meat bites

Ingredients

- ½ can crab meat

- 4 ounces cream cheese

- ¼ cup cream

- ½ tbsp. lemon juice

- 1 tbsp. onion (finely chopped)

- 1 tbsp. red bell pepper (finely chopped)

- 1 tbsp. celery (finely chopped)

- ¼ cup mustard (dry)

- ¼ tsp. salt

Method

1. Preheat the oven to 350 degrees Fahrenheit.

2. Drain the crabmeat from the can and clean the meat well. Remove any bits of shell.

3. Make sure that the cream cheese is left to soften at the room temperature.

4. Take a large mixing bowl and add the ingredients to the bowl.

5. Bake miniature tarts in the oven. Add the crab mixture to the tarts and place them in the oven for ten minutes at 350 degrees Fahrenheit. Serve hot.

Taco Bites

Ingredients

- 1 tbsp. butter

- ½ yellow onion (chopped)

    o   cloves garlic (minced)

- ½ pound beef (ground)

- 2 ounces can green chilies

- 1 tsp. cumin (ground)

- 1tsp. chili powder

- ½ tsp. coriander (ground)

- ½ cup sour cream

- 1 cup Cheddar Cheese (grated)

Method

1. Preheat the oven to 350 degrees Fahrenheit.

2. Take a medium skillet and place it on a medium flame. Add the butter to the skillet and wait till the butter melts.

3. Add the onions to the skillet and sauté. Make sure that they have become soft.

4. Add the beef to the skillet and cook till it is brown.

5. Add the spices to the skillet along with the green chilies from the pan and cook for five minutes.

6. Reduce the heat and add the cheese and the cream to the skillet and simmer for a few minutes.

7. Continue to stir the mixture for a few minutes till the cheese has melted and has mixed well into the beef.

8. Pre bake some piecrusts and add the mixture to the crusts.

9. Bake the crusts in the oven with the beef for a few minutes until the cheese is bubbling.

Zucchini Pancakes

Ingredients

- 2 Zucchinis (shredded)

- 2 cups almond flour

- 3 eggs

- 2 tsp. dried basil

- 2 tsp. dried parsley

- Salt and Pepper to taste

- 3 tbsp. Butter

Instructions

1. Take a small mixing bowl and add the shredded zucchini, along with the basil and the almond flour.

2. Mix the ingredients well. Once the zucchini is coated well with the flour, add the parsley, pepper and the salt to the bowl.

3. Ensure that the taste of the mixture is well balanced.

4. You can make close to 10 patties from the mixture that you have just made.

5. Take a large non – stick sauce pan and place it on a medium flame.

6. Add one teaspoon to the pan. Once the butter has started warming up, add the patties and cook them one after the other.

7. Ensure that you remove the patty off the pan when it is brown on both sides.

Creamy Chocolate Smoothie

Ingredients

- 8 ounces almond milk (preferably unsweetened)

- ½ packet artificial sweetener

- 2 ounces heavy cream

- ½ scoop Whey Chocolate isolate powder

- ¼ cup crushed ice (this could increase depending on your liking)

Method

1. Blend all the ingredients together in the processor or a blender until it is smooth. You could increase the amounts of each ingredient if you want to since it is low on carbohydrates.

Low Carb Mojito

Ingredients

- 10 mint leaves with their stems attached

- 2 tbsp. low carb sugar syrup

- 4 ounces light rum

- 2 limes

Method

1. Dice the mint leaves finely.

2. Take a tall glass and add the mint leaves to the low carb sugar. Mix the two well.

3. Cut the two limes in half and remove the seeds.

4. Squeeze the juice from both limes into the glass and mix well.

5. Add the rum and stir.

6. You could either add just ice or add club soda as well to increase the taste.

Spicy tea

Ingredients

- 2 regular tea bags

- 1 cup water

- 1 cup grass fed milk

- 2 cloves

- 2 cardamom pods

- ½ stick cinnamon

- 2 teaspoons sweetener

Method

1. Start by adding the water to a pan and allow it to boil.

2. Bash the spices a little to help them release their flavor.

3. Add them to the water and allow them to infuse their flavor.

4. Add the tea bags to it the water and wait for them to infuse.

5. Meanwhile, heat the milk with the sweetener.

6. Remove the tea bags and strain the spicy liquid into a glass.

7. Add in the sweet milk and mix until well combined.

8. Serve the tea hot.

Cleansing tea

Ingredients

- 2 green tea bags

- 2 teaspoons cumin seeds

- 1 teaspoon turmeric powder

- 1 teaspoon honey

- Water

Method

1. Add the water to a saucepan and add in the cumin and turmeric.

2. Allow it to come to a boil.

3. Add in the tea bags to a cup.

4. Pour the water over the tea bag and allow it to infuse.

5. Remove the tea bag after a while.

6. Add in honey to it and give it a good mix.

7. Serve the tea hot.

Flower infused black tea

Ingredients

- 1 large hibiscus flower

- 2 roses

- 1 black tea bag

- 1 cup water

Method

1. Start by heating the water in a pan.

2. Meanwhile, remove the petals of the hibiscus and also that of the roses.

3. Add them to the boiling water and allow the flavor to infuse.

4. Add the tea bag to a cup.

5. Add the flower water to it and allow the tea to infuse for a while.

6. Serve hot.

Fruit infused water

Ingredients

- 1 pitcher water

- 1 cucumber

- 1 large orange

- 1 lemon

- ½ cup mint leaves

Method

1. Start by cutting the orange and lemon into thin slices.

2. Peel and cut the cucumber into cubes.

3. Add the cucumber to the jug and use a muddler to bruise it.

4. Now add in the oranges and lemon to it and give it a mix.

5. Chop the mint leaves roughly and add to the pitcher.

6. Give it a good mix such that all the flavors combine.

7. Serve this water instead of regular water.

Cooling water

Ingredients

- 1 cup coconut water

- 1 cup plain water

- ½ cup rose petals

- Crushed ice

- Mint to sprinkle

Method

1. Start by adding the plain water to a pan and allow it to boil.

2. Add in the rose petals and let it infuse its flavor and color.

3. Boil it for 10 minutes.

4. Use a strainer to strain the petal water.

5. Pour it into a jug.

6. Add in the coconut water and give it a good mix.

7. Add the crushed ice to glasses and then pour the liquid into it.

8. Serve with some mint on top.

Papaya smoothie

Ingredients

- 1 ripe papaya

- 1 ripe banana

- 1 cup almond milk

Method

1. Start by cutting the papaya in half and remove some of the seeds from it.

2. Use a sharp knife to cut out pieces from it.

3. Add it to the blender.

4. Cut the banana into small pieces and add to the blender.

5. Add in the milk and whizz until smooth.

6. Serve as is or chill in the freezer and serve.

Coffee with a twist

Ingredients

- 1 teaspoon coffee powder

- 1 cup almond milk

- 2 tablespoon grass fed butter

- 1 tablespoon sweetener

Method

1. Start by heating the milk.

2. Add the butter to a cup along with the coffee powder and give it a good mix.

3. Add the sweetener to the milk and allow it to dissolve in the heat.

4. Pour it into the coffee cup and give it a good mix.

5. Serve hot.

Strawberry and coconut shake

Ingredients

- 1 cup coconut milk

- 2 tablespoons coconut cream

- ½ cup fresh strawberries, chopped

- Mint to garnish

Method

1. Start by chopping the strawberries.

2. Add the coconut milk to a blender along with the chopped strawberries.

3. Whizz until everything well combines.

4. Add it to a glass.

5. Mix in the coconut cream.

6. Garnish with mint leaves on top and serve.

Green apple soda

Ingredients

- 2 green apples

- 1 cup cold soda

Method

1. Start by peeling the apples and cut them into small pieces.

2. Add them to a jug or pitcher.

3. Use a muddler to bruise them a little.

4. Pour in the soda and give it all a good mix.

5. Pour it into a glass and serve cold.

Lemon and ginger drink

Ingredients

- 2 large lemons

- 2 inch ginger stick

- 2 tablespoons honey

- 1 cup soda

Method

1. Start by squeezing the lemons into a glass.

2. You can also remove some zest to add later.

3. Grate in the ginger.

4. Add the soda and mix in the honey.

5. Serve cold.

Cheddar Pepper Biscuits

Ingredients

- 5 cups almond flour

- 12 ounces Colby jack cheese (shredded)

- 10 tbsp. butter

- 16 ounces cream cheese

- 4 large eggs or 6 medium eggs

- 4 tsp. ground pepper

- 2 tsp. baking soda

- 2 tsp. Xanthan gum

- 2 tsp. sea salt

Method

1. Take a cookie sheet and grease it well. Line it with parchment paper if you do not want to grease it.

2. Then preheat the oven to300 degrees Fahrenheit.

3. Process the shredded cheese and one cup of the almond flour in a food processor till they have blended well and are granular. Keep this aside.

4. Take a large mixing bowl. Add the butter and the cream cheese to the bowl and place. You have to melt the better a little. Once it has melted, mix the butter and the cheese together. Make sure that the mixture is smooth and glossy.

5. Add the eggs to the mixture and continue to whisk. Make sure that the mixture is smooth and glossy.

6. Add the pepper, the Xanthan gum, baking soda and the salt to the mixture.

7. Add the remaining almond flour and cheese mixture to the egg mixture and whisk well.

8. Once the ingredients have blended well, add the almond flour that is left and continue to fold the mixture well. You have to ensure that the dough has formed.

9. Take a tablespoon and scoop the dough and place it on the cookie sheet. Keep the cookies one inch apart. If you

want you could flatten the dough a little to ensure that you have a smooth biscuit.

10. Place the cookie sheet in the oven and bake for thirty minutes. You will need to leave the biscuits in till they have a golden brown color.

11. Remove the biscuits from the oven and cool to room temperature. You can serve it with a glass of milk.

Chapter 11:
Recipes for Desserts

Lemon Cheesecake
Ingredients

- 16 ounces cream cheese (softened at room temperature)

- 4 ounces heavy cream

- 2 tsp. Stevia glycerite

- 2 tsp. Splenda (or any other artificial sweetener which is low in carbohydrates)

- 2 tbsp. lemon juice

- 2 tsp. vanilla essence or flavoring

Method

1. Add all the ingredients in a large mixing bowl.

2. Whisk them well until it has a consistency that is pudding like.

3. Spoon the batter into small cups and leave it in the refrigerator to set.

Chocolate Cherry Cheesecake

Ingredients

- 16 ounces cream cheese (softened at room temperature)

- 4 ounces heavy cream

- 2 tsp. Stevia glycerite

- 2 tsp. Splenda (or any other artificial sweetener which is low in carbohydrates)

- 2 tbsp. Dutch processed cocoa powder

- 2 tbsp. Sugar free cherry syrup

Method

1. Add all the ingredients in a large mixing bowl.

2. Whisk them well until it has a consistency that is pudding like.

3. Spoon the batter into small cups and leave it in the refrigerator to set.

Caramel chocolate chip muffin

Ingredients

- 3 cups almond flour

- ¼ cup xylitol

- 1 tsp. baking soda

- 1 tsp. salt

- 1 tsp. Xanthan gum

- 3 large eggs (crack the eggs in a glass bowl and beat them lightly.)

- 1 ½ cup sour cream

- 3 tbsp. butter (melt the butter.)

- 2 tsp. Stevia glycerite

- 1 cup Caramel dip (ensure that you buy low carb)

- 2 cups Chocolate chips

Method

1. Preheat the oven to 300 degrees Fahrenheit.

2. Line a muffin tray with paper liners or grease them well.

3. Take a medium bowl and add the xylitol, almond flour, baking soda, xanthan gum and salt and whisk them together.

4. Take a smaller bowl and add the eggs and beat them well. Add the butter, sour cream and the stevia glycerite and mix well.

5. Add the egg mixture to the flour mixture. Stir well and ensure that the mixture is smooth and glossy.

6. Fill each cup with the mixture. Do not fill it up to the brim.

7. Leave the muffin tray in the oven for thirty minutes. Make sure that the muffins are brown and firm to touch.

8. Remove the muffins to cool. This will make it easier for you to remove them from the paper without too much pressure.

9. Store the muffins in an airtight container and leave them in the refrigerator.

Coconut Cream Macaroons

Ingredients

- 2 large eggs (only remove the whites)

- ¼ tsp. cream of tartar

- 1/8 tsp. salt

- ½ tsp. vanilla

- 1 cup erythritol

- 8 ounces dried coconut (unsweetened, dried and finely shredded)

- 4 ounces cream cheese (soften at room temperature)

- 1 ounce heavy cream

- 1 ounce Sugar free white chocolate syrup

- 1 ounce chocolate chips

Method

1. Preheat the oven to 300 degrees Fahrenheit.

2. Take a cookie sheet and line it with parchment paper.

3. Take a large mixing bowl and beat the egg whites, the tartar and the salt using an electric mixer or a blender.

4. Add the erythritol only one tablespoon at a time and keep beating the mixture until the mixture is smooth.

5. Add the coconut and keep folding it well.

6. Add the cream cheese and the heavy cream and smoothen the mixture. Add the syrup and mix the ingredients well.

7. Add the coconut mixture in thirds until it has combined well. Add the chocolate chips and fold the dough well.

8. Use a small scoop and add the coconut mixture to the sheet.

9. Leave them in the oven to cook for thirty minutes. Once they have been cooked for that long, leave them in the oven to dry for another thirty minutes.

10. Transfer back to the rack to cool.

Rich chocolate muffin

Ingredients

- 3 cups almond flour

- 2 cups heavy cream

- 3 large eggs

- 1 cup melted butter

- 1 cup xylitol

- 2 tsp. vanilla extract

- 2 tsp. baking soda

- ½ tsp. salt

- 1 cup chocolate chips (ensure that the brand you choose has low carbohydrates)

Method

1. Preheat the oven to 300degrees Fahrenheit.

2. Keep the muffin covers in each hole of the muffin pan.

3. Take a small bowl and add the cream and the almond flour. Whisk the two ingredients together.

4. Add the eggs one at a time and keep stirring till the mixture has become smooth.

5. Add the butter, baking soda, sweetener, flavoring and the salt to the bowl. Mix all the ingredients together.

6. Add the chocolate to the bowl and stir the ingredients together till they are distributed evenly.

7. Take the mixture and place it in each of the muffin holes. Bake the cupcakes for thirty minutes. Leave them in the oven till they are golden brown.

8. Let them cool down. Serve them with butter.

Sago pudding

Ingredients

- 1 cup sago pearls

- 2 cups almond milk

- 2 tablespoons honey

- 2 tablespoons chopped pistachios

- 2 tablespoons chopped walnuts

- 2 tablespoons chopped almonds

- 2 tablespoons ghee or clarified butter

Method

1. Start by soaking the pearls in enough water and wait for them to swell up.

2. Meanwhile, add the milk to a saucepan and add in the honey.

3. Allow it to come to a boil.

4. Now add in the sago pearls to it and allow it to thicken.

5. In a small pan add the ghee and allow it to heat up.

6. Now toss in the chopped nuts and allow them to brown.

7. Add it to the pudding and mix.

8. Serve hot or cold.

Chickpea flour fudge

Ingredients

- 1 cup chickpea flour

- 1//2 cup ghee or clarified butter

- 1 teaspoon cardamom powder

- 1 cup sweetener of your choice

- 1 cup water

Method

1. Start by adding the clarified butter to a pan and ad in the chickpea flour.

2. Allow it to brown.

3. Add the water and sweetener to a pan and allow it to form a 2-string consistency.

4. Add the powdered cardamom to the chickpea flour.

5. Add the sweetener water to the chickpea and mix until well combined.

6. The mixture should start to thicken.

7. Once done, remove the mix on a greased plate and allow it to cool.

8. Once cool, you can use a sharp knife to cut it into diamonds.

Cold Melon soup

Ingredients

- 1 large melon

- 1 cup melon water

- 1 tablespoon honey

- 2 tablespoon mint leaves

Method

1. Cut the lemon and use ice cream scoop to remove scoop sized pieces.

2. Add the melon water to a bowl along with the honey and give it a good mix.

3. Add in the melon pieces and place it in the fridge for an hour.

4. Sprinkle the fresh mint leaves on top and serve as a dessert.

Lentil pudding

Ingredients

- 1 cup split yellow lentils

- 2 cups coconut milk

- ½ cup coconut flesh

- 1 tablespoon cardamom powder

- ½ cup sweetener of your choice

Method

1. Start by soaking the yellow lentils in enough water overnight.

2. The next day, boil it and cook it until soft.

3. Put half of it in a grinder and make a smooth paste.

4. Add the coconut milk and coconut paste to a blender and make a smooth paste.

5. Add it to a pan and allow it to boil.

6. You can add in a little water to thin it.

7. Add in the boiled and ground lentil paste to it along with the sweetener.

8. Allow it to thicken.

9. Add in the cardamom powder and serve the pudding hot.

Easy pops

Ingredients

- Any low carb cake of your choice, homemade or store bought

- 1 cup mixed fruit juice

- ½ cup low carb chocolate chips

Method

1. Start by crumbling the cake into a large bowl.

2. Add in enough fruit juice to make it pliable. Don't add too much though, you should have a binding consistency.

3. Add the chocolate chips to a double boiler and melt away.

4. Make small cake crumb balls and attach it to a lollipop stick.

5. Now dip it in the melted chocolate and freeze for an hour.

6. Your easy cake pops are ready to serve.

Banana cake

Ingredients

- 1 cup almond flour

- 2 teaspoons baking powder

- 2 teaspoons vanilla extract

- ½ cup milk

- ½ cup butter

- 1 cup sweetener of your choice

- 3 bananas

- ¼ cup walnuts

Method

1. Preheat the oven to 350 degrees Fahrenheit.

2. Start by adding the baking powder into the almond flour and sieve it to combine well.

3. Add the butter to the milk and beat until well combined.

4. Add in the sweetener and mix well.

5. Add in the vanilla extract and the flour and form a smooth batter.

6. Mash the bananas and add it to the mix.

7. Grease a baking tray.

8. Add the walnuts to the better and add it to the baking tray.

9. Bake for 30 minutes or until a skewer inserted in the center comes out clean.

10. Cut and serve.

Peach ice cream

Ingredients

- 2 cups heavy whipping cream

- 1 cup half & half

- ¼ cup water

- 1/3 cup Sweetener of your choice

- 2 large peaches

- Mint sprigs

Method

1. Start by adding the peach to a blender and create a smooth paste.

2. Add in the whipping cream and half and half and whip further.

3. Add in the sweetener and water and make a smooth paste out of everything.

4. Prepare the ice cream maker.

5. Add in the mix to the maker and follow the instructions provided to you.

6. Serve the ice cream with a mint sprig on top.

Chocolate chip cookies

Ingredients

- 5 tablespoons coconut flour
- 2 cups almond flour
- ½ teaspoon baking soda
- 1 egg
- 1 teaspoon vanilla extract
- ¼ cup butter
- ⅓ cup sugar free chocolate chips
- ½ cup sweetener

Method

1. Start by preheating the oven to 350 degrees Fahrenheit.

2. Mix the flour, coconut flour, baking powder and sieve together.

3. Add the butter, vanilla, egg and sweetener to a bowl and beat it until well combined.

4. Add in the flour to it and mix well.

5. Add in the chocolate chips to it and mix until well combined.

6. Use a scoop to pick the right sized amount of the batter on a tray.

7. Place it in the oven and bake for 15 to 20 minutes.

8. Serve warm.

Chapter 12:
The Sample Plan!

This chapter leaves you with a sample plan that you can use to test whether or not the diet is for you.

Day 1

    Breakfast – Chocolate Raspberry Protein Shake

    Lunch – Apple and Spinach Salad

    Snack – Crab meat bites

    Dinner – Glazed Pork Tenderloin

Day 2

    Breakfast – Bacon and Egg

    Lunch – Decadent keto Meatloaf

    Snack – Taco Bites

    Dinner – Creamy chicken salad

Day 3

    Breakfast – Pumpkin Pancakes

    Lunch – Chicken Guadalajara

    Snack – Zucchini pancakes

    Dinner – Chicken, Tomato and Bacon Salad

Day 4

Breakfast – Baked Bacon and Eggs

Lunch – Baked Salmon

Snack – Rich chocolate muffin

Dinner – Egg Salad

Day 5

Breakfast – Onion and cheese quiche

Lunch – Herb Baked Salmon

Snack – Low Carb mojito

Dinner – Keto Italian meatballs

Day 6

Breakfast – White chocolate almond protein shake

Lunch – Keto Italian meatballs left over from dinner

Snack – Lemon cheesecake

Dinner – Pizza with sausages

Day 7

Breakfast – Onion and cheese quiche

Lunch – Pizza with sausages (leftover from dinner)

Snack – Chocolate Cherry cheesecake

Dinner – Zucchini pancakes with cheddar pepper biscuits

Conclusion

Thank you for purchasing the book.

The book tells you everything you need to know about the ketogenic diet. The first chapter of the book talks about basics of the ketogenic diet. The benefits of the diet are innumerable and some of them have been mentioned to you in this book. You have also been given delicious recipes for breakfast, lunch and dinner. There are a few recipes for desserts as well!

The last chapter of the book comprises of a seven-day plan that you could use to test whether or not the diet is for you. You have to ensure that you do not quit! If you find yourself losing weight quickly, you will be happy about continuing with the diet. But, when you find yourself not losing weight, you will tend to lose interest in the diet and will quit. You have to keep pushing yourself to stick to the diet. You can take a break if you choose to for a day, but ensure that you do not binge eat.

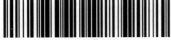

Made in the USA
San Bernardino, CA
28 September 2016